born.
yogis

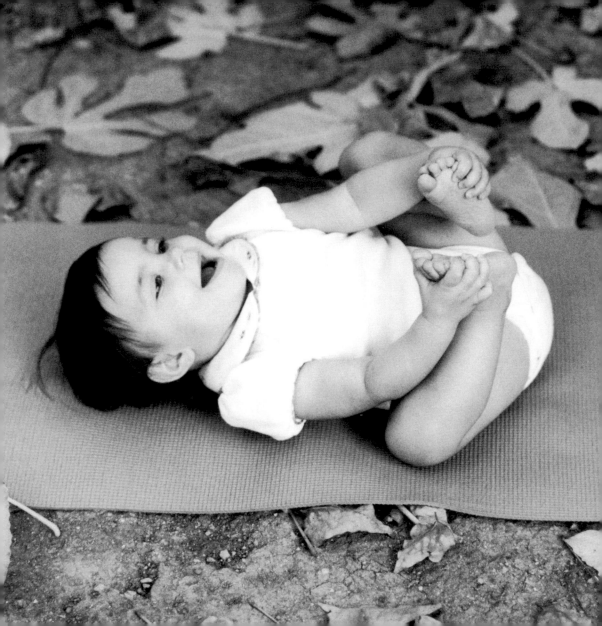

born.
yogis

Susie Arnett and Doug Kim
Foreword by Gurmukh Kaur Khalsa

RODALE

Printed in China
Rodale Inc. makes every effort to use acid-free ♾, recycled paper ♻.
B.K.S. Iyengar's quotations on pages vi, 6, 20, 25, 39, 41, 45, 49, 53, 54, 63, 83, 88, and 90
are reprinted with his permission.

Book design by Christina Gaugler

Library of Congress Cataloging-in-Publication Data

Arnett, Susie.
    Born yogis / Susie Arnett and Doug Kim ; foreword by Gurmukh Kaur Khalsa.
       p.   cm.
    ISBN-13 978–1–59486–275–5 hardcover
    ISBN-10 1–59486–275–3 hardcover
    1. Hatha yoga for infants.   2. Hatha yoga for infants—Pictorial works.   I. Kim,
Doug, photographer.   II. Title.
RJ133.7.A76   2005
613.7'046—dc22   2005015188

Distributed to the trade by Holtzbrinck Publishers

2   4   6   8   10   9   7   5   3   1   hardcover

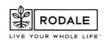

RODALE
LIVE YOUR WHOLE LIFE™

We inspire and enable people to improve their lives and the world around them

For more of our products visit **rodalestore.com** or call 800-848-4735

ACKNOWLEDGMENTS

Many people participated in the birthing of *Born Yogis*. First of all, we'd like to thank Suzanne Balaban, whose support, encouragement, and skill in introducing our book to the publishing world were invaluable.

Also, we'd like to thank Margot Schupf for making a home for our book at Rodale. Jennifer DeFilippi was instrumental in helping us flesh out our concept and make the book a reality. Thanks, also, to Sara Sellar for guiding us with her sure hand and to Christina Gaugler for the charming design of our book.

Daniel Greenberg's generosity with his time and wisdom also made a big difference in helping us navigate the publishing waters.

Without Dennis Dalrymple guiding us through the negotiating process, we would have quickly lost our path and been left to wander aimlessly.

The yogis who helped us with the research are Michelle Broussard, Annmarie Solo, and Britta Bushnell.

Our thanks also to Mr. B.K.S. Iyengar, whose inspiring words bring our images to life.

There were many mothers, such as Melissa Oliver, Hiro Zeoli, and Dhari Thein, who helped by schlepping their babies to our shoots or by opening their homes to us.

Kathy Wu designed a stunning mock-up of the book when we had only three photos and an idea. And where would we be without Noureddine El-Warari, who printed all of the photographs in this book and whose hands create such beautiful images out of the darkness.

Finally, a big thank you to our families for their love and inspiration.

Liberation is in the little things, here and now.

—B.K.S. Iyengar

FOREWORD

One day, in my Mommy and Me yoga class, a little girl went into a perfect Downward-Facing Dog pose. We all watched, cheering her on. Like all children, she was born with the innate knowing of this age-old practice. The ancient scriptures say that babies perform the 108 postures of yoga while in the womb. One of our jobs as teachers and parents is to remind our young ones of what they already know and help them develop this inner wisdom.

The photographs in this book inspire, helping us to realize yoga comes very naturally to every one of us, young and old. *Born Yogis* is simple, pure, and uplifting, and it will make you smile, even laugh. I thoroughly enjoyed reading it, and I know it will be another way to bring forth the light in our little ones, as well as inspire joy in us all. God bless the children.

Peace to all, light to all, love to all,

Gurmukh Kaur Khalsa
Director, Golden Bridge Yoga
Los Angeles, California
May 2005

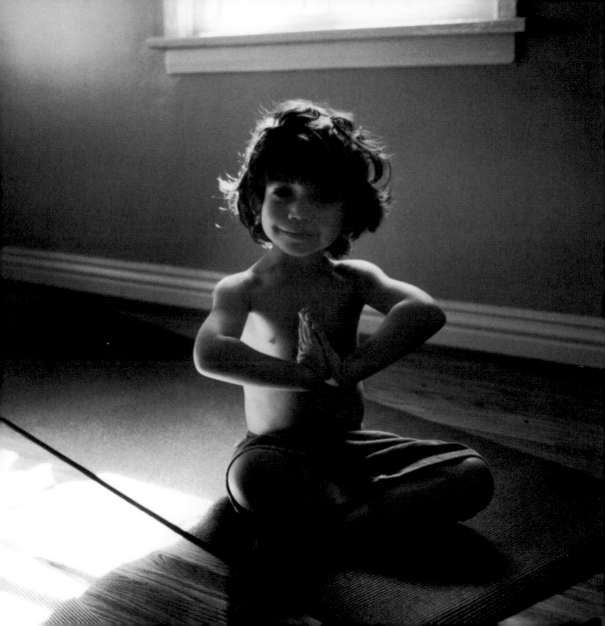

INTRODUCTION

Babies are born yogis.

At every stage of development, they naturally curl and bend into a variety of asanas that would make a master yogi green with envy. When learning how to crawl, they arch their torsos up into Cobra. And just before they walk, they spend weeks crossing rooms in Downward-Facing Dog. Even while sleeping, they unconsciously tuck into the aptly named Baby Pose.

These poses build coordination and strengthen the muscles necessary for babies to grow. Yoga is an innate exercise on a child's journey to becoming vertical, as it is our conscious practice along a journey to self-realization. Whether it's flexibility we strive for or deep, deep focus (there's no one more present than an infant gazing into her mother's eyes), yoga helps us regain what we were born with and what we gradually lose as we age.

Noticing that a baby naturally performs yoga is one thing; getting these poses to occur in front of a camera is quite another story. The photographs in this book are captured moments: natural and candid fractions of a second when the lighting, expression, and pose all work together. Most images reflect poses and moves that were completely spontaneous; the only staged element was the placement of the yoga mat in the proper light.

In shooting the photos for this book, an enormous amount of patience and perseverance was required. The payoff to this waiting and the many rolls of exposed film were these wonderful and lyrical moments that could never have been anticipated. On the second shoot with Myles, he suddenly fell into an amazingly tight Backbend Pose, which his mother had never seen him do before. He promptly twisted into two more Backbends before running off to play.

Zane, the baby performing Mountain Pose, was crawling around the deck of a house when he suddenly stood up, raising his arms into the air in exultation. His parents squealed, because this was his first time standing. That $\frac{1}{125}$ of a second, that little slice of magic never to be repeated, is just one of the many moments forever captured within these pages.

Because the age-old spirit of yoga inhabits babies so completely, we have reached back into many ancient yogic texts, from the original yoga treatise, *Bhagavad Gita,* to Patanjali's *Yoga Sutras,* to find passages that illuminate and complement the mood of the photos.

The accompanying text is also culled from modern writings such as the works of B.K.S. Iyengar. Whether written in 500 BC or today, meditative or exultant, playful or quiet, these words are intended to open our eyes to the depth of spirit that exists in our children. They are not only yogis, they are our gurus as well.

This collection mirrors the sequence of a Sun Salutation, which is traditionally performed at the beginning of the day. We hope that as you travel through the following pages, these baby gurus—these born yogis—will carry you a little further toward enlightenment.

—SUSIE ARNETT AND DOUG KIM

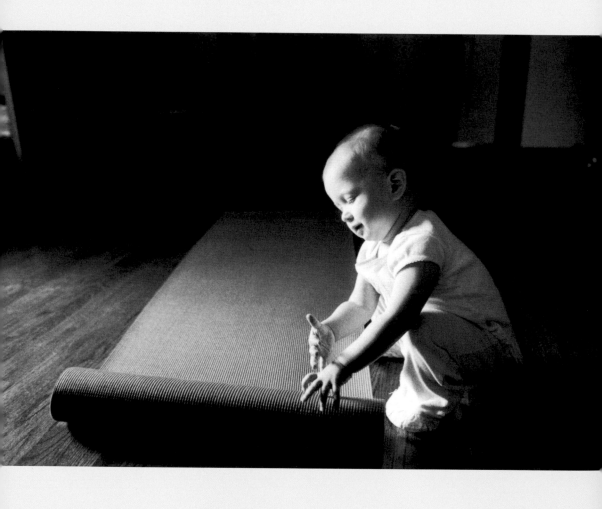

Find a quiet retreat for the practice of Yoga,

sheltered from the wind, level and clean,

free from rubbish, smouldering fires, and ugliness,

and where the sound of waters and the beauty of the place

help thought and contemplation.

—*The Upanishad*

Margaret
16 months

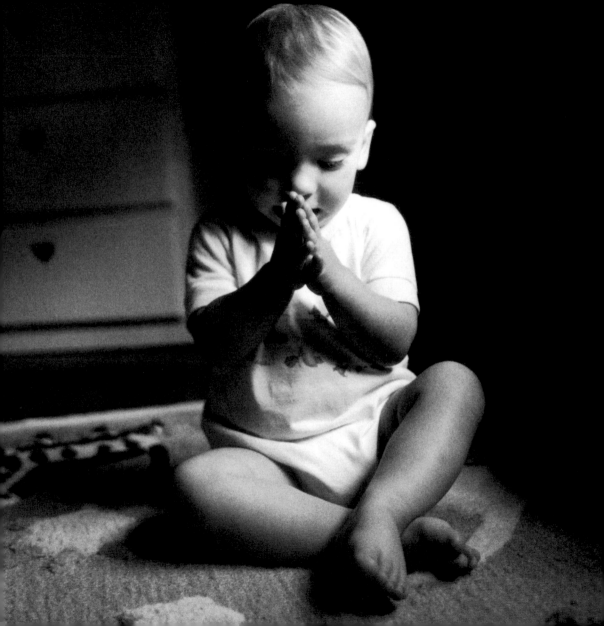

Sukhasana
Easy Pose

When the five senses and the mind are still,

and reason itself rests in silence,

then begins the path supreme.

This calm steadiness of the senses

is called Yoga.

—*The Upanishad*

Kadin
13 months

Tadasana
Mountain Pose

The first fruits of the practice of Yoga are health,

little waste matter, and a clear complexion;

lightness of the body, a pleasant scent, and a sweet voice;

and an *absence of greedy desires.*

—THE UPANISHAD

Zane
14 months

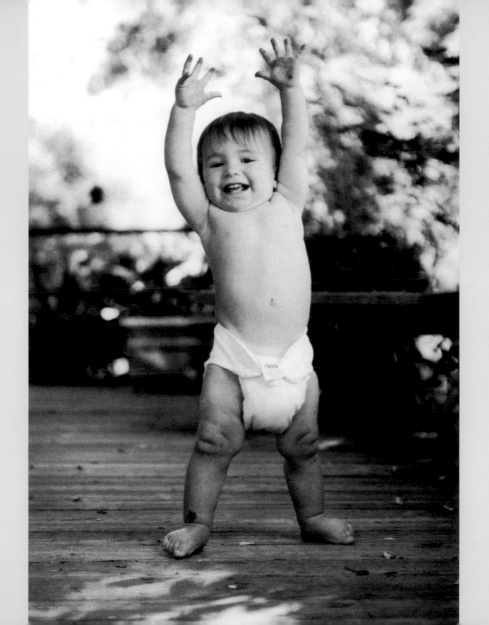

Uttanasana
Forward Bend

This is a boon to people who get excited quickly, as it **soothes** the brain cells. After finishing the asana, one feels **calm** and **cool,** the eyes start to glow, and the mind feels at **peace.**

—B.K.S. IYENGAR

Callie
16 months

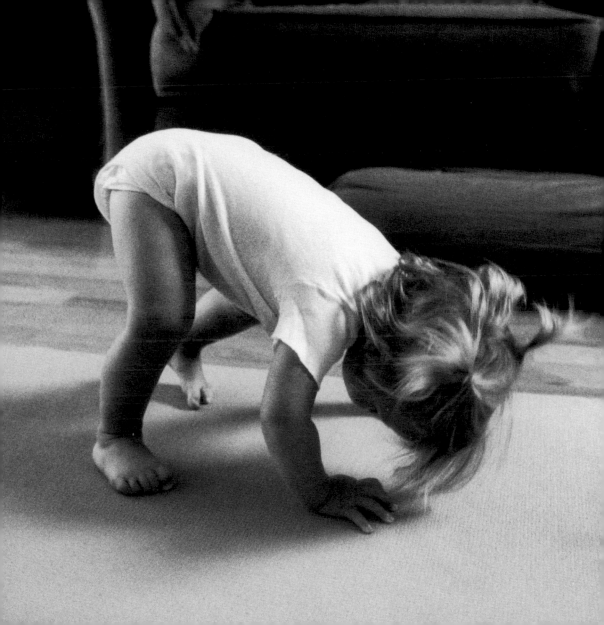

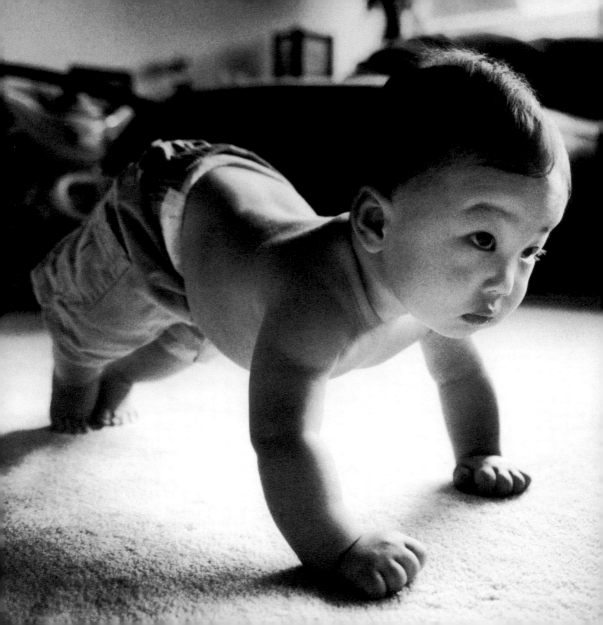

Chaturanga Dandasana
Four-Limbed Staff Pose

When the Yogi has FULL POWER

over his body composed of the elements

of earth, water, fire, air, and ether,

then he obtains a new body of

SPIRITUAL FIRE which is

beyond illness, old age, and death.

—*The Upanishad*

Mason
7 months

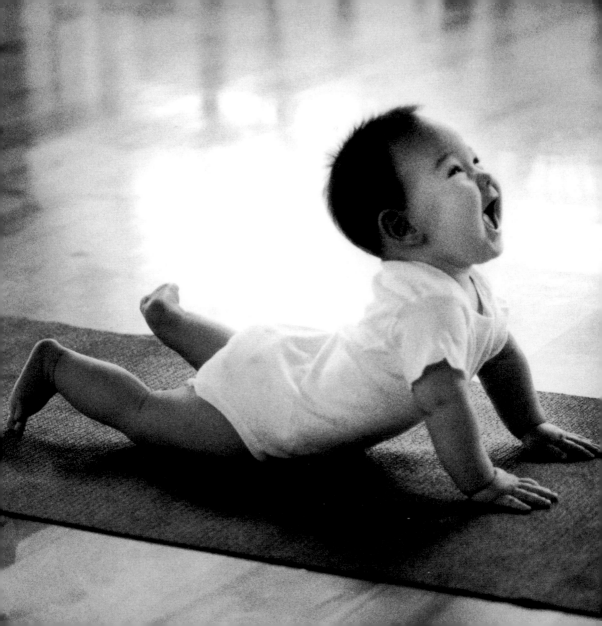

Bhujangasana I
Cobra

The body should touch the ground from the navel down to

the toes. Placing the palms on the ground, one should raise

the head and shoulders like a serpent. This is said to raise

the body temperature and remove diseases of all kinds, as

well as awaken the "serpent power."

—*Gheranda Samhita*

Ely
7 months

Adho Mukha Svanasana
Downward-Facing Dog

Do not consider your body a mere lump of flesh. . . .

IT IS A NOBLE INSTRUMENT.

In it are situated all holy places, gods, mantras,

and the source of all extraordinary powers in this world. . . .

GOD DWELLS IN THE BODY.

—SWAMI MUKTANANDA

Everly
8 months

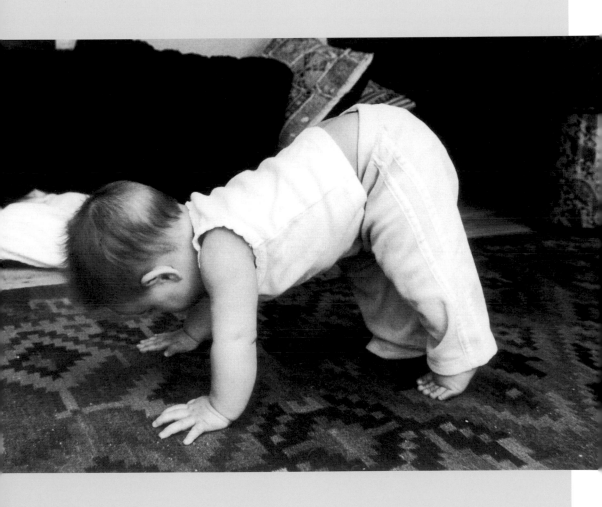

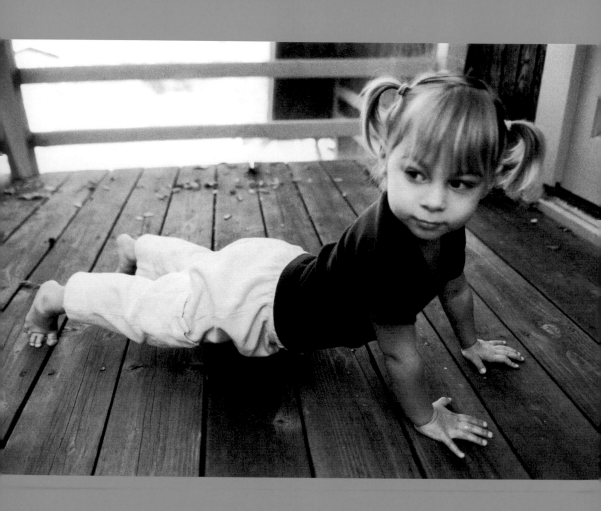

Urdhva Mukha Svanasana
Upward-Facing Dog

The body always wears away like an unbaked clay

pot placed in water. Therefore, one should cultivate

bodily fitness by tempering it with the fire of Yoga.

—GHERANDA SAMHITA

Cheyanne
32 months

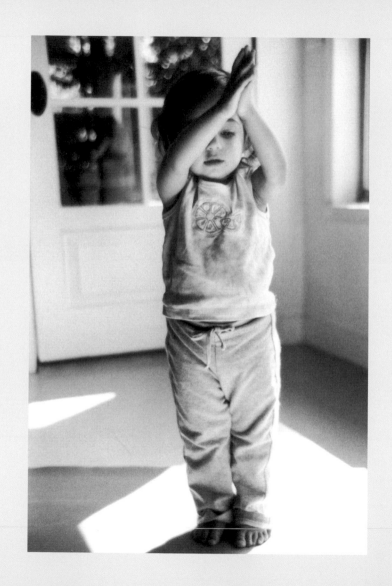

Tadasana
Mountain Pose

By day, it is the sun which shines,

at night the moon shines forth.

A warrior shines in his armour,

and a Brahmin shines in meditation.

—DHAMMAPADA

Isabela
20 months

Trikonasana
Triangle Pose

The meaning of

our *SELF* is not to be found

in *SEPARATENESS* from God and others,

but in the ceaseless realization of yoga, of *UNION*.

—RABINDRANATH TAGORE

Cosmo
28 months

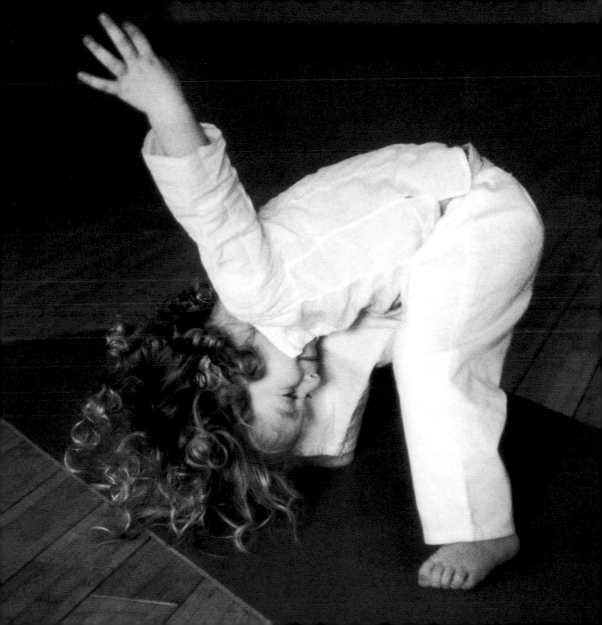

Virabhadrasana I
Warrior I

Stand erect,

or you cave in the very Self.

—B.K.S. IYENGAR

Leon
36 months

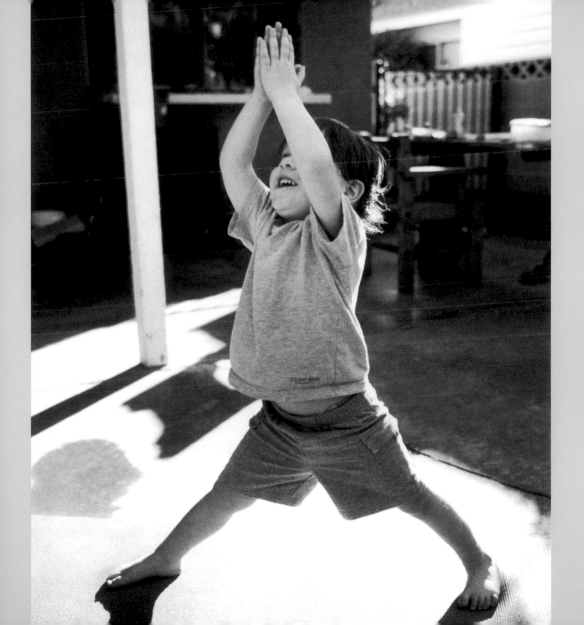

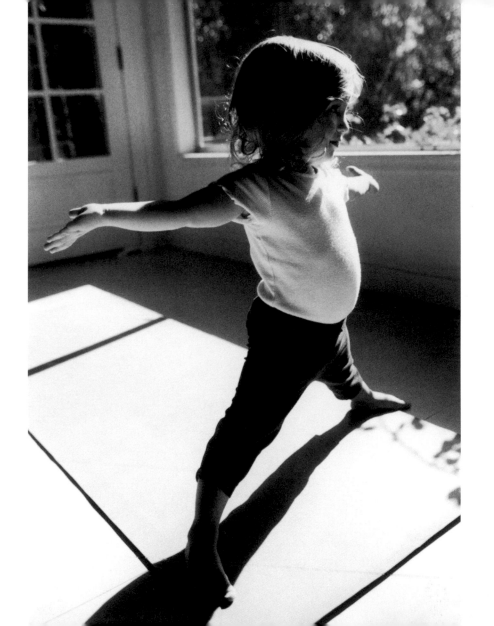

Virabhadrasana II
Warrior II

Like to a rock that's of one mass,

And by the wind unshook,

E'en so, by praise or blame,

Unmoved are the wise.

—*Dhammapada*

Isabela
26 months

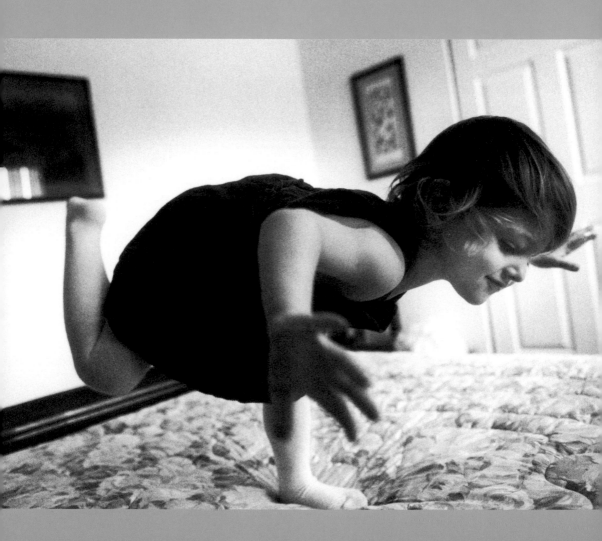

Virabhadrasana III
Warrior III

Balance

is the gift of the Creator.

—B.K.S. Iyengar

Alexandra
31 months

Utkatasana
Chair Pose

When you look into another's eyes,

what you see is the Self,

fearless and deathless.

That is the Higher Spirit,

Brahman, the Supreme.

—*THE UPANISHAD*

Margaret
16 months

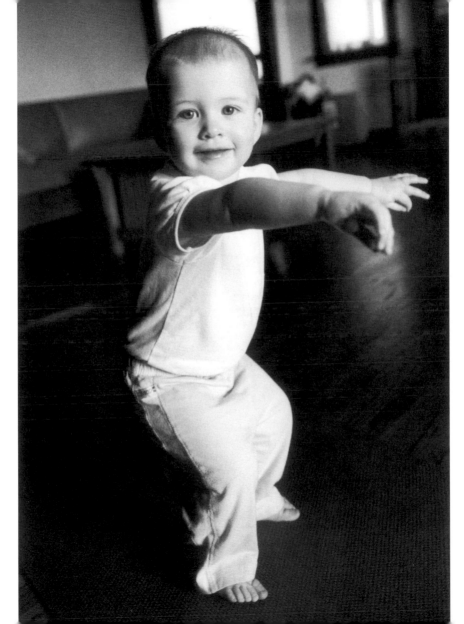

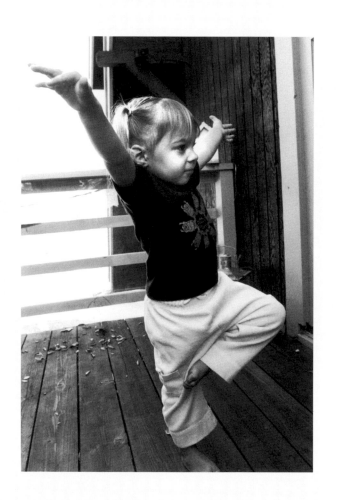

Vrksasana
Tree Pose

All duties, wealth, enjoyments, liberation,

All people and objects in the world as well;

Everything, in the eyes of a yogi,

Is like the [illusory] water in a desert mirage.

—*Avadhuta Gita*

Balasana
Child's Pose

As a tortoise contracts its limbs into the middle of the shell,

so the yogin should withdraw the senses into himself.

—*Goraksha-Paddhati*

Left to right: **Zachary and Isabel**
Both 17 months

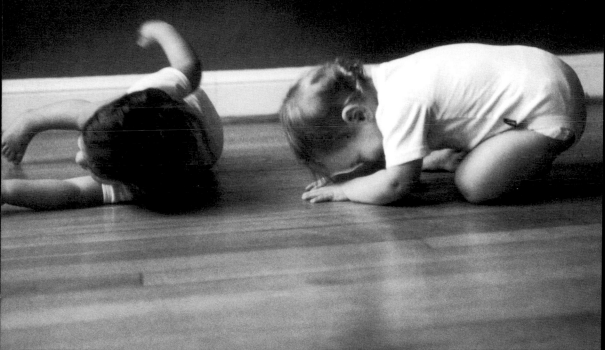

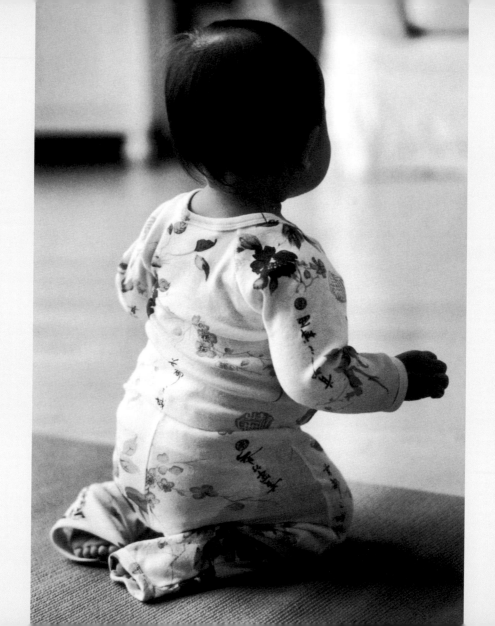

Virasana
Hero Pose

Seated in a solitary place,

free from desires and with senses controlled,

one should meditate free of thought

on that one infinite Self.

—SHANKARA

Taryn
13 months

Suptavirasana
Reclining Hero Pose

From my *light*

The body and the world arise.

—ASHTAVAKRA GITA

Ford
32 months

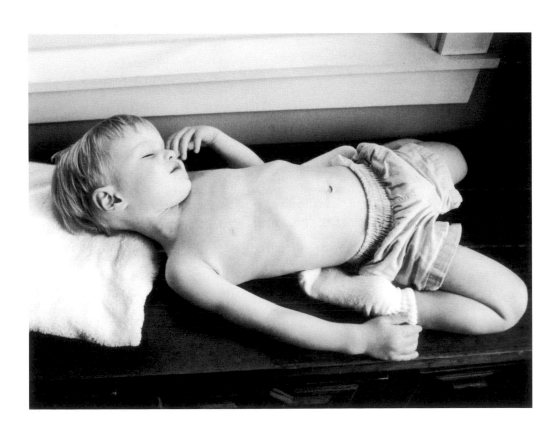

Matsyasana
Fish Pose

Health is *Wealth*.

Peace of Mind is *Happiness*.

Yoga Shows the Way.

—SWAMI VISHNU-DEVANANDA

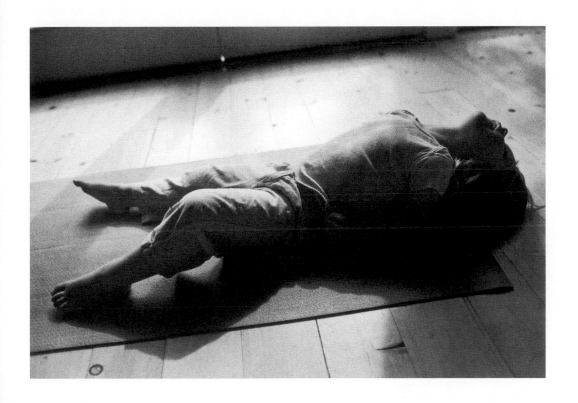

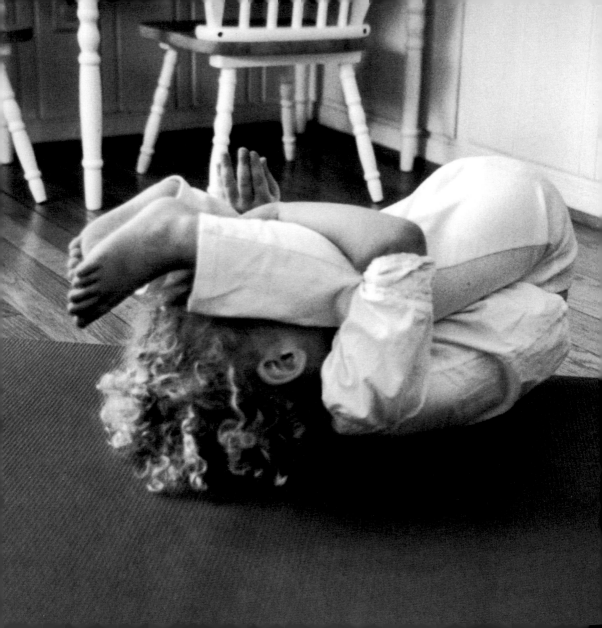

Halasana
Plough

Any holy person is a yogi.

Any yogi is a holy person.

—B.K.S. IYENGAR

Emerson
34 months

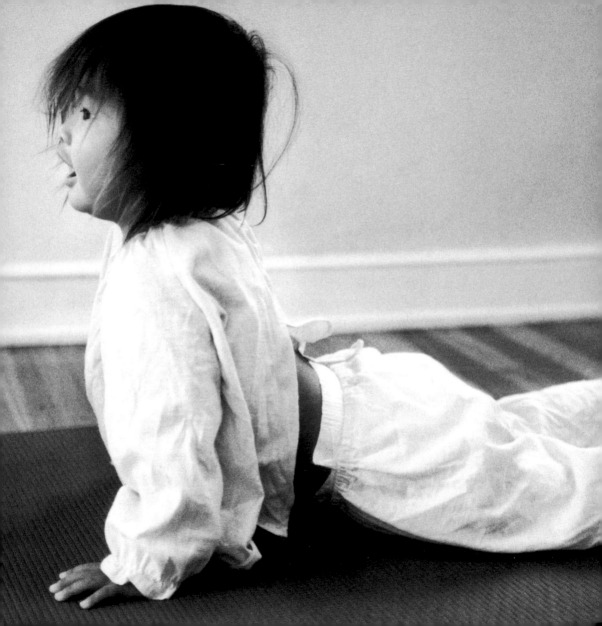

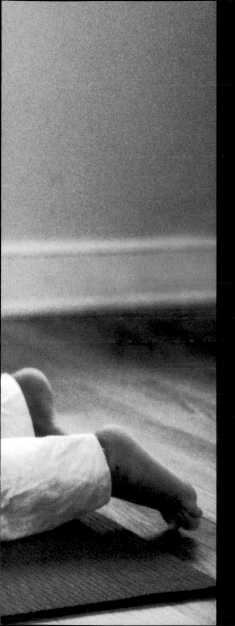

Urdhva Mukha Svanasana
Upward-Facing Dog Pose

In asanas,

we are CHANTING

with our bodies.

—B.K.S. IYENGAR

Maisie
25 months

Shalabhasana
Locust Pose

Asanas make one FIRM,

FREE from maladies,

and *light of limb.*

—HATHA-YOGA-PRADIPIKA

Maya
5 months

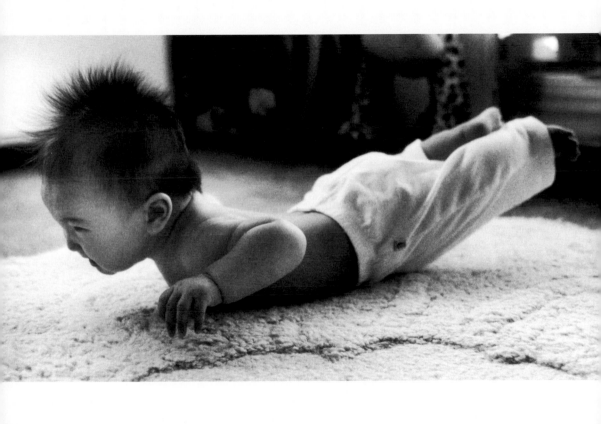

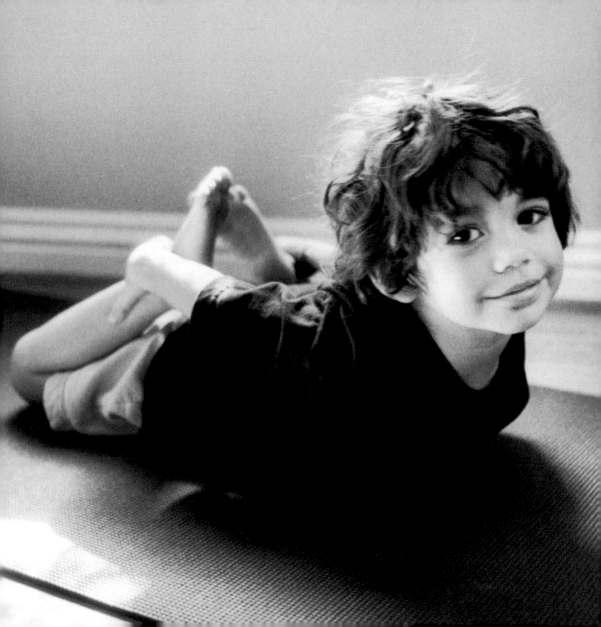

Dhanurasana
Bow Pose

Body is the bow,

asana is the arrow,

and soul is the target.

—B.K.S. IYENGAR

Asher
35 months

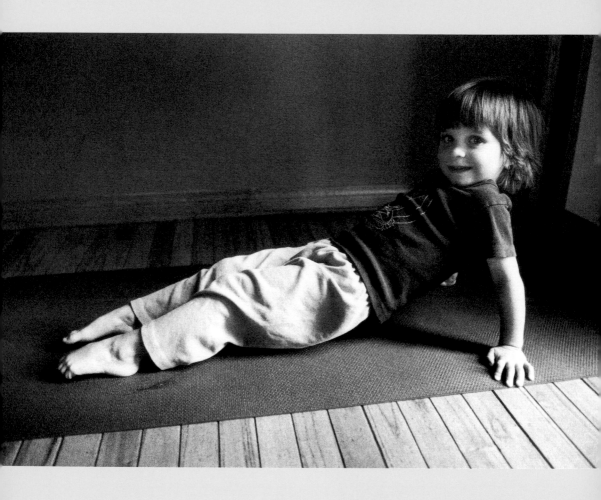

Purvottanasana
East Stretch Pose

My Guru told me;

that child, which is you even now, is your real self.

Go back to that state of pure being,

where the *I Am* is still in its purity

before it got contaminated with

This I Am or *That I Am.*

—RAMANA MAHARSHI

Tydeman
35 months

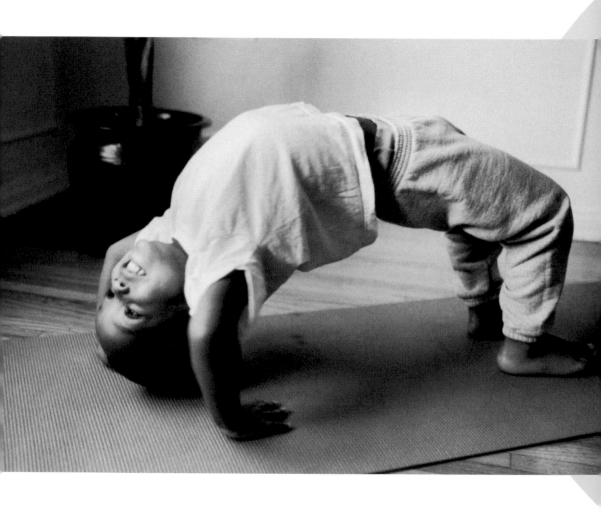

Urdhva Dhanurasana
Upward-Facing Bow Pose

Yoga is like *music*.

The *rhythm* of the body,

the *melody* of the mind,

and the *harmony* of the soul

create the *symphony of life*.

—B.K.S. Iyengar

Myles
29 months

Sirsasana
Headstand Pose

He who practices

the headstand for

3 hours daily

CONQUERS TIME.

—*The Upanishad*

Lily
29 months

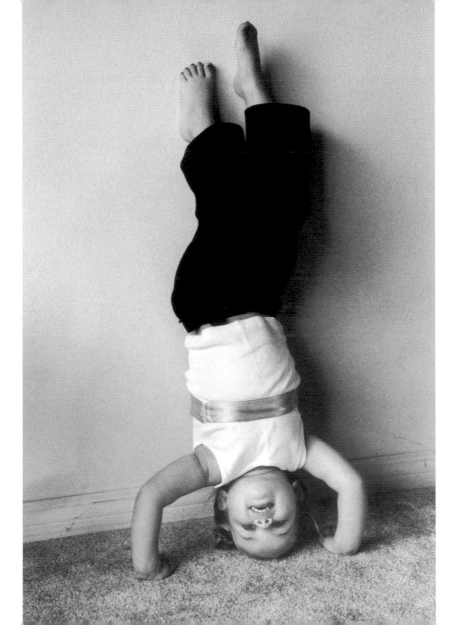

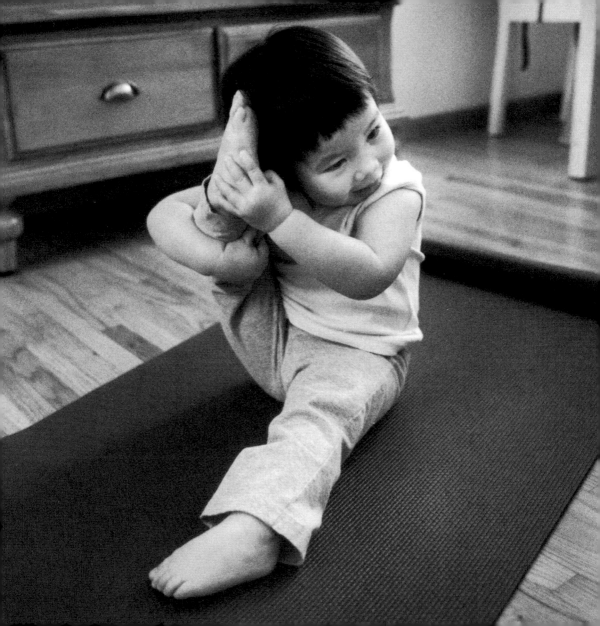

Eka Pada Sirsasana
Foot-behind-the-Head Pose

It is the quest of the soul,

the spark of divinity within us,

which is the very purpose of yoga.

—B.K.S. IYENGAR

Kelly
22 months

Upavistha Konasana
Wide-Angle Seated Forward Bend Pose

The body is the temple of the spirit.

Let the temple be clean through Yoga.

—B.K.S. IYENGAR

Eden
8 months

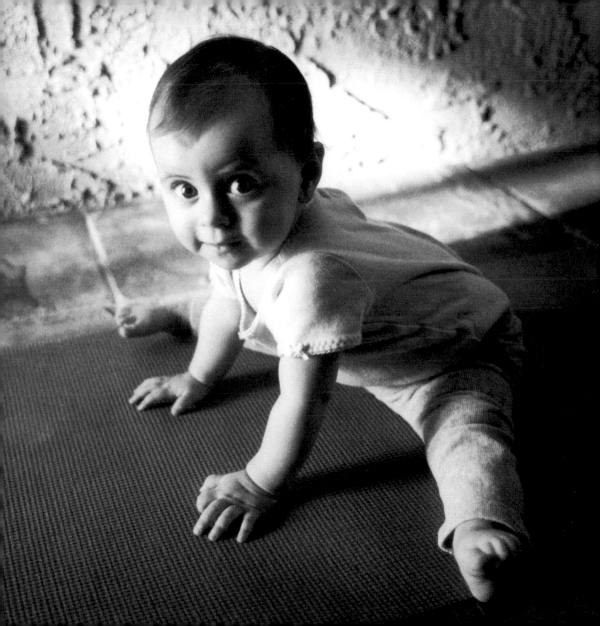

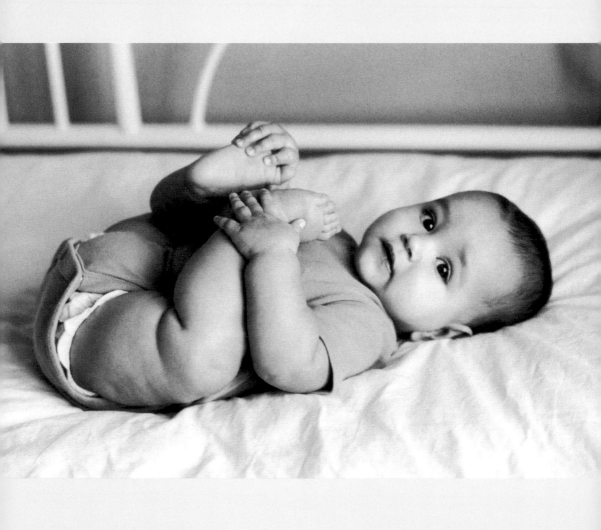

Happy Baby Pose

The sage contemplated the outer elements of earth, sun, fire,

and water, and the inner elements of eye, ear, mind, bones,

skin, and muscles, and he discovered . . .

everything is holy!

—THE UPANISHAD

Nathan
5 months

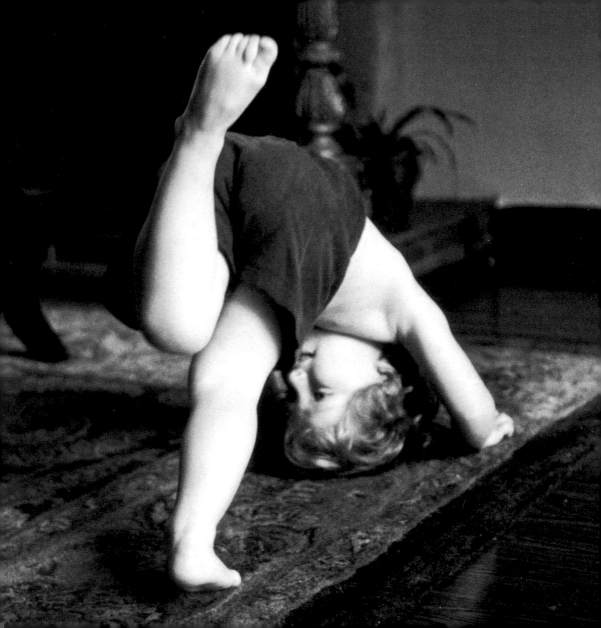

Adho Mukha Svanasana
Downward-Facing Dog

As by learning the alphabet,

one can, through practice, master all the sciences,

so by thoroughly practicing first physical training,

one acquires the knowledge of Truth.

—GHERANDA SAMHITA

Tobias
36 months

Navasana

Boat Pose

No matter that I have not expressed it yet,

it is in me. All knowledge is in me,

all power, and *all freedom.*

—SWAMI VIVEKANANDA

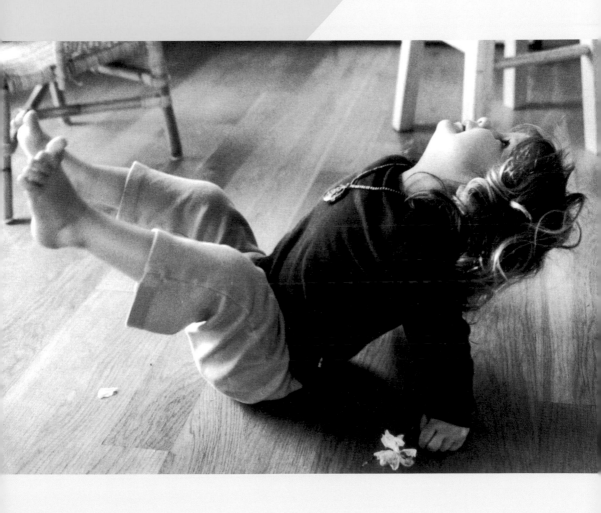

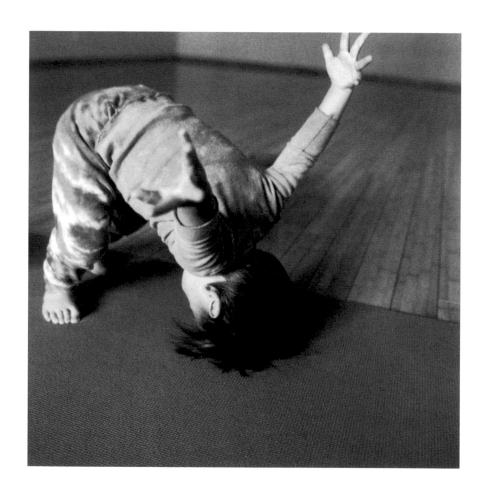

Prasarita Padottanasana
Wide-Legged Forward Bend

Yoga is the music of the soul.

So do continue, and the

gates of the soul will open.

—B.K.S. IYENGAR

Miles
26 months

Nakrasana
Crocodile Pose

By constant meditation, one forgets the world,

then in sooth, the Yogi obtains wonderful powers.

—SHIVA SAMHITA

Erin
8 months

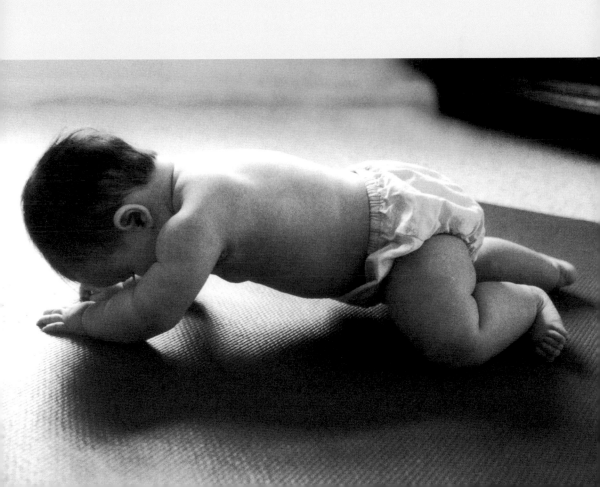

Ugrasana
Fearful Pose

Stretch both legs joined and holding firmly

the feet with the hands, place the head on the knees.

This is called the Fearful posture, which stimulates

the fire of the *life breath*.

—SHIVA SAMHITA

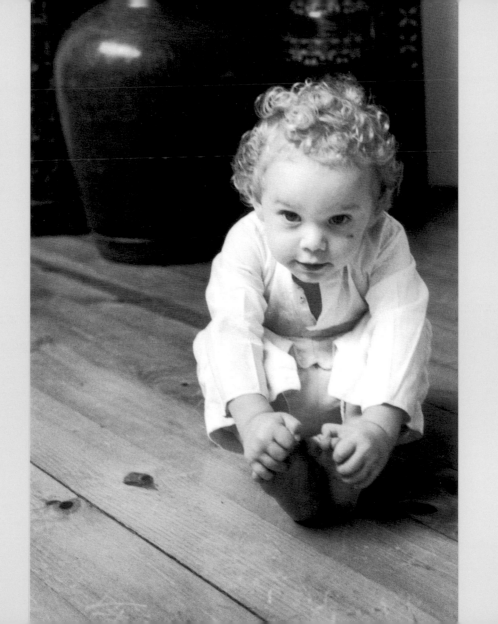

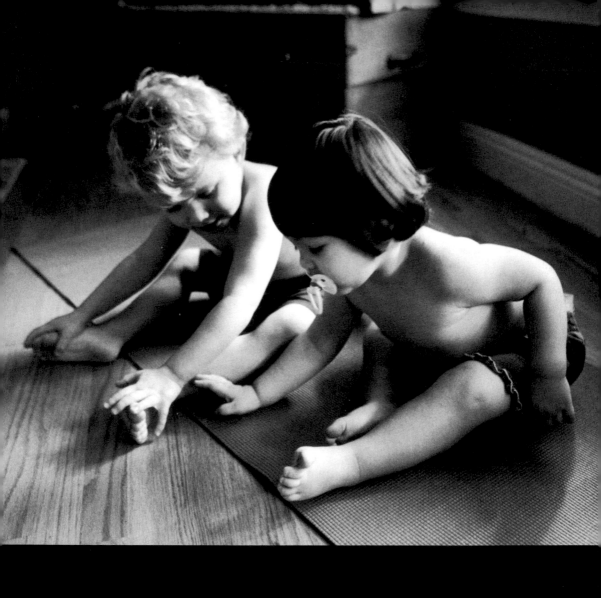

Paschimottanasana
Forward Bend Pose

The sages know this to be practice:

being DEDICATED to one thing,

REFLECTING upon it,

TALKING about it with one another,

and UNDERSTANDING it.

—YOGA-VASISHTHA

Left to right: Robbie and Megan
30 months and 22 months

Paschimottanasana
Forward Bend Pose

Yoga is the restraint

of the thought-waves

of the mind.

—*YOGA SUTRAS*

Aidan
11 months

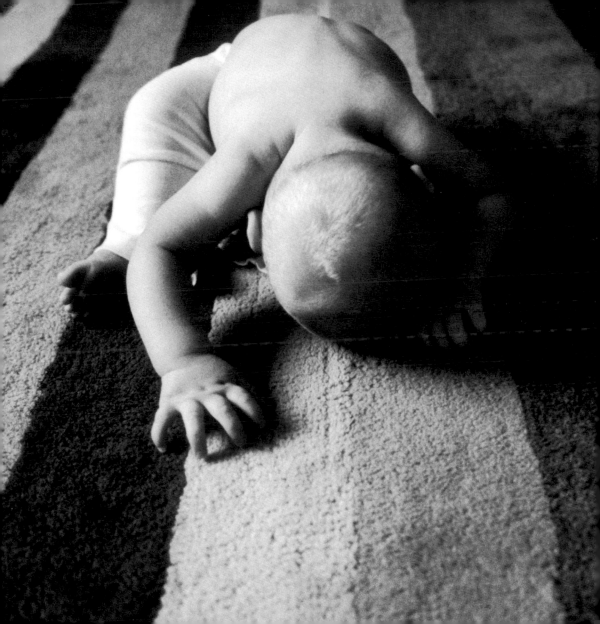

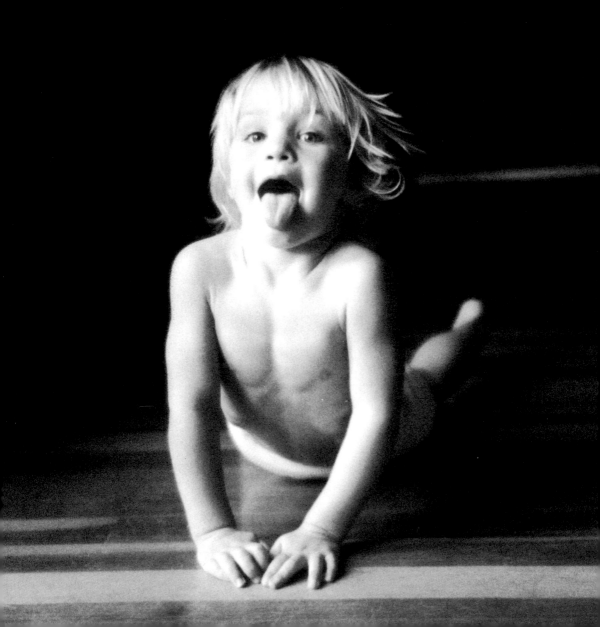

Bhujangasana II
Sphinx Pose

. . . O goddess, difficult to find is a guru

who lights up everything like the sun.

—*Kula-Arnava-Tantra*

Forrest
23 months

Simhasana
Lion Pose

Stand as a rock; you are indestructible.

You are the Self, the God of the universe. Say:

"I am Existence Absolute, Bliss Absolute,

Knowledge Absolute, I am He."

—Swami Vivekananda

Max
36 months

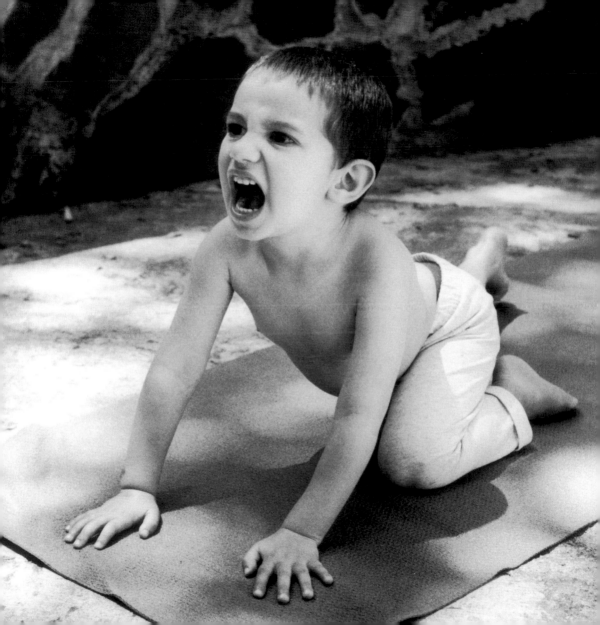

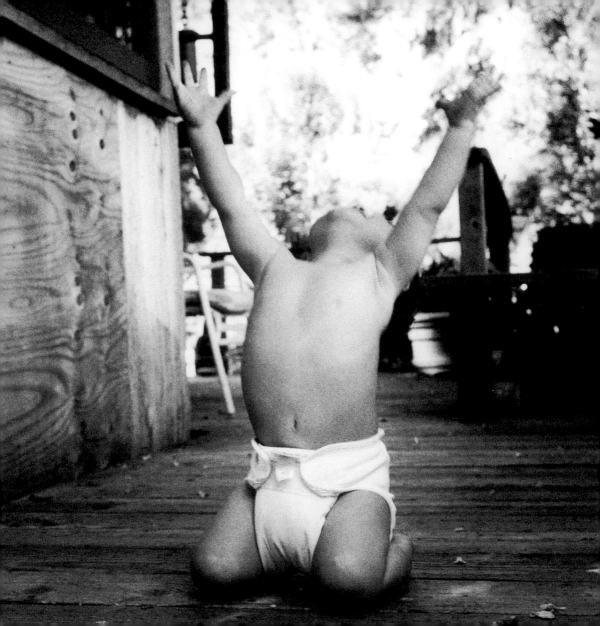

Virasana
Hero Pose

I have neither Guru nor initiation;

I have no discipline, and no duty to perform.

Understand that I'm the formless sky;

I'm the self-existent Purity.

—A<small>VADHUTA</small> G<small>ITA</small>

Zane
14 months

Viralasana
Cat Pose

Success in Yoga is not obtained by the near theoretical reading

of sacred texts. Success is not obtained by wearing the dress

of a yogi or a sanyasi (a recluse), nor by talking about it.

Constant practice alone is the secret of success.

Verily, there is no doubt of this.

—HATHA-YOGA-PRADIPIKA

Roman
7 months

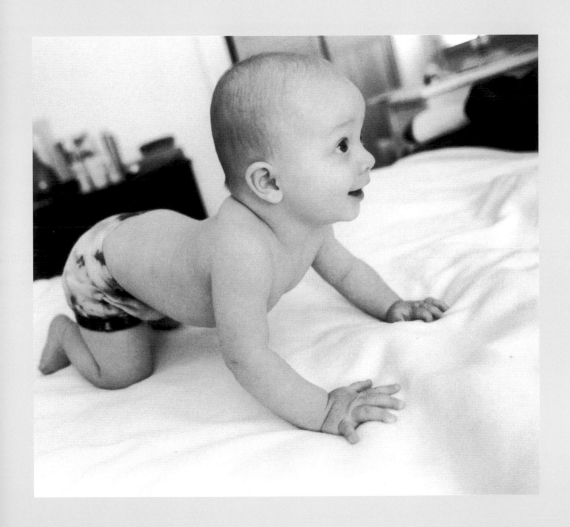

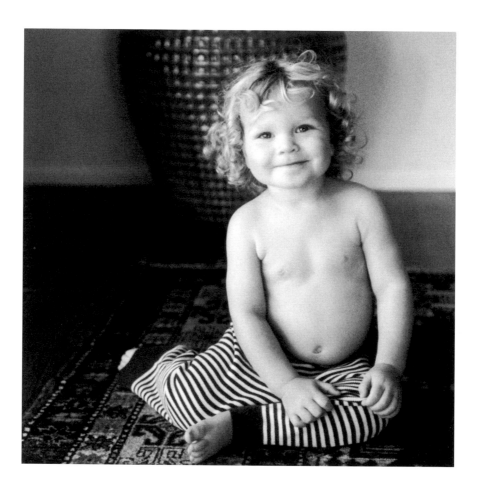

Bharadvajasana
Seated Twist Pose

Those seekers of Yoga,

with PURE MIND AND HEART,

discover the Atman within themselves.

—*Bhagavad Gita*

Aidan
23 months

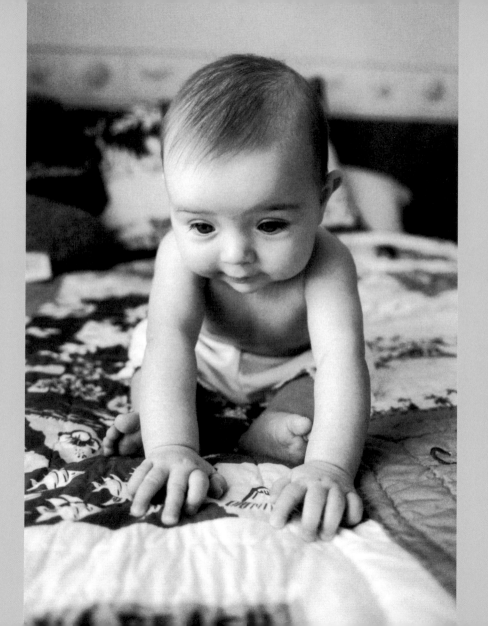

Paschimottanasana
Forward Bend Pose

In each pose,

there should be repose.

B.K.S. IYENGAR

Vanessa
4 months

Happy Baby Pose

Sow love, *reap peace* . . .

sow meditation, *reap wisdom.*

—SWAMI SIVANANDA

Emi
4 months

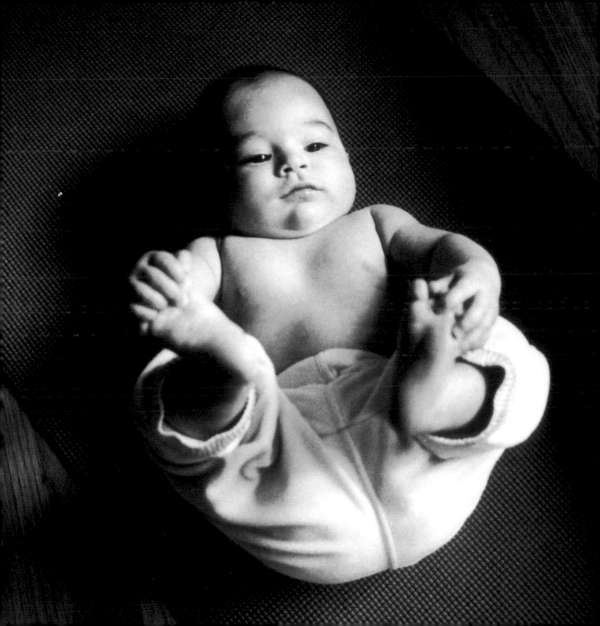

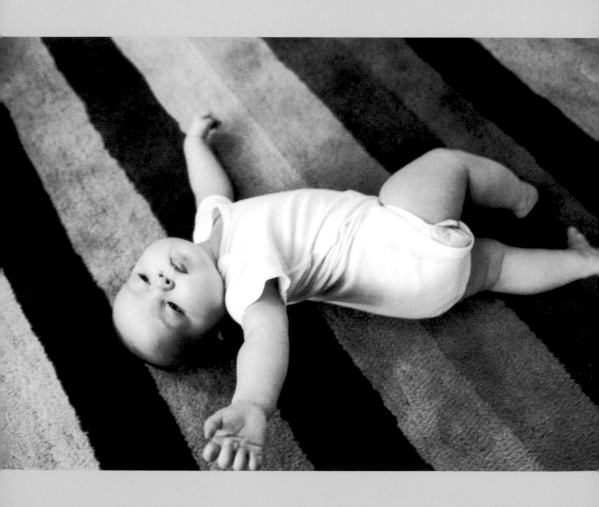

Jathara Parivartanasana
Revolved Abdomen Pose

The practice of yoga will not lead you to purity;

Silencing the mind will not lead you to purity;

The Guru's instructions will not lead you to purity.

That purity is your Essence;

It's your very own Consciousness.

—Avadhuta Gita

Erika
7 months

Supta Baddha Konasana
Reclining Bound-Angle Pose

You must savor the fragrance of the posture.

—B.K.S. IYENGAR

Jackson
4 months

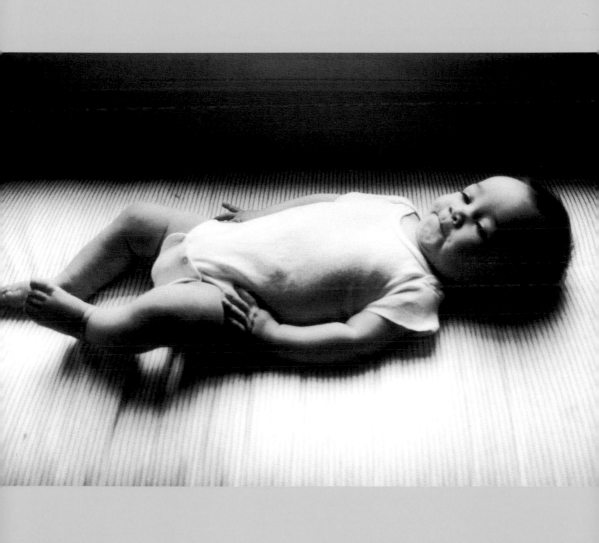

Jathara Parivartanasana
Revolved Abdomen Pose

Each movement is my mantra.

—B.K.S. IYENGAR

Logan
10 months

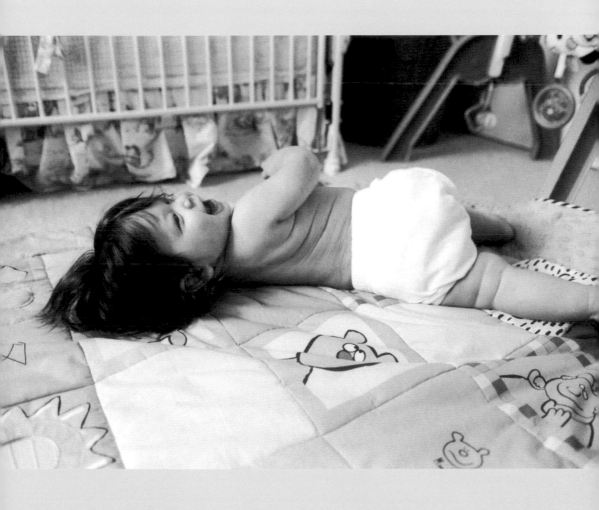

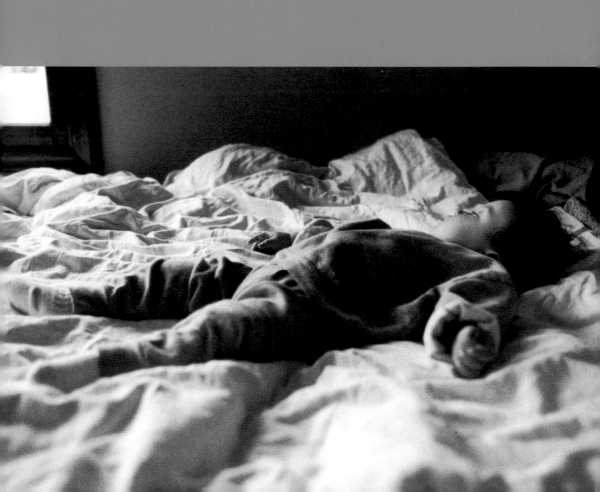

Mrtasana
Corpse Pose

Lying flat on the ground like a corpse

is called the Mrtasana (the Corpse posture);

this posture destroys fatigue

and quiets the agitation of the mind.

—GHERANDA SAMHITA

Cole
9 months

Sukhasana
Easy Pose

Through the practice of yoga,

and understanding the paths

of darkness and light,

you reach the greatest state of all,

coming home to the Divine love

that lives in your heart.

—*BHAGAVAD GITA*

Emma Jane
27 months

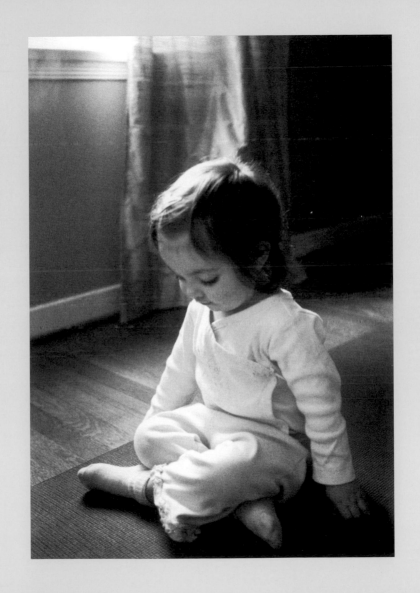

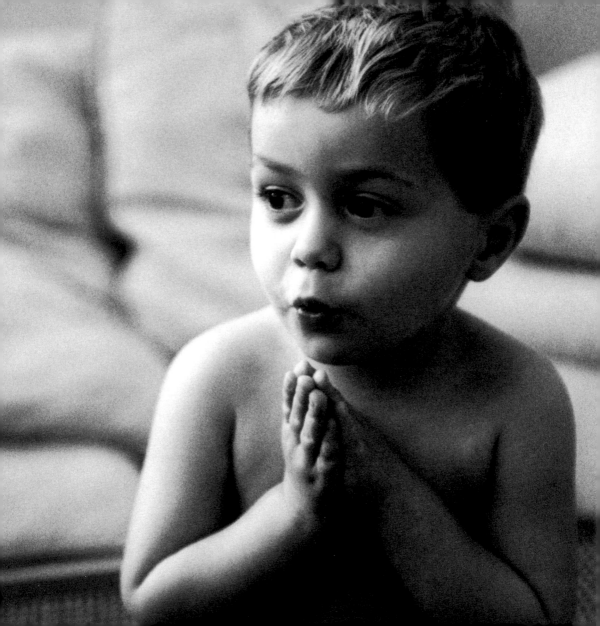

Pranayama
Breath Control

OM is spirit. Everything is OM.

OM is the beginning of the ancient chants.

The priests start with OM, the teachers start with OM.

The student murmuring OM seeks the spirit

and finds it in the end.

—*The Upanishad*

Bruno
34 months

JUST AS A SEED BECOMES A TREE,

with branches, leaves, flowers, and fruit, so within

Her own being, Chiti becomes animals, birds, germs,

insects, gods, demons, men, and women. I could

see this radiance of Consciousness, resplendent and

utterly beautiful, silently pulsating as supreme ecstasy

within me, outside me, above me, below me.

—SWAMI MUKTANANDA

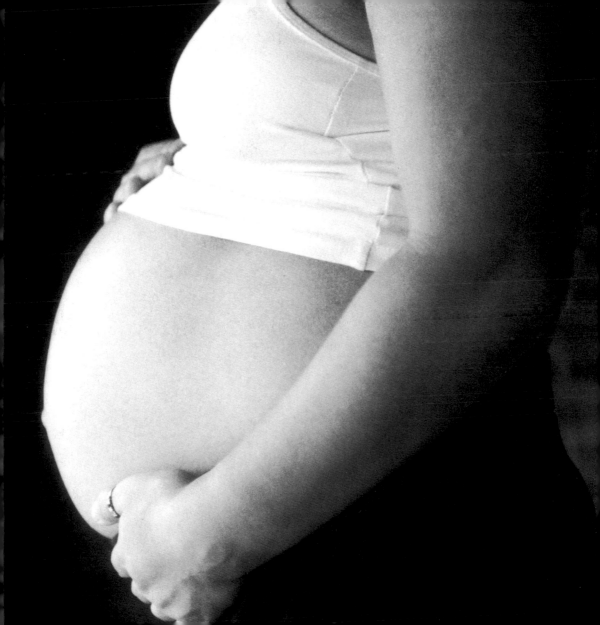

namaste